W9-CZV-285

Disclaimer: This book should not be considered medical advice. The author is not a medical professional. Any advice given is the opinion of the author and should be checked with a medical professional.

ISBN: 978-0-9710230-3-1

Published by Orsorum
New York, New York USA

ꝏꝏꝏ

Thank You

The list of people that I have to thank on this journey is long and would take a book in its own right but I wanted to acknowledge a few key individuals.

Thank you to my wife who is my rock and champion.

Thank you to **Dr. Geoffrey Westrich** and the incredible team at **Hospital for Special Surgery** for providing such amazing care.

Thank you to **Justin Horwath** and the team at **SPEAR Physical Therapy** in Chelsea for helping me reconnect to the muscles that took some time off.

Thank you to the Facebook group, **Hip Replacement Total Support Group.** You gave me knowledge when

I sought it, encouragement when I needed it, and cheered when I celebrated the small wins.

Diary of a Hippie

A Real-Life Journal of What to Expect During a Total Hip Replacement

About This Book

When the pain got too much to bear and I started blocking out time to have the procedure, I began my quest to find out all I could about what I would be going through. My surgeon was excellent in providing information, as were the articles on websites like The Mayo Clinic, and Hospital for Special Surgery, but they were clinical and general overviews on the actual procedure, or about why it needed to be done, but not about what I would experience.

I looked for information about what I would GO THROUGH. What would it be like the week after. I wanted information from those who had gone through the forest and come out the other side. I didn't find much. And so I decided to keep a journal of the time leading up to the operation and in the days, weeks, and months after so that I might post some trail markers for others to follow. Everyone's experience is different and we all heal at our own pace. This was mine. Hopefully it will help you with yours.

The format is a journal entry about what I was going through on a particular day, with an inspirational quote related to the entry. At the bottom of each entry is a "What You Need to Know" block which summarizes the entry and gives you the important information in a concise manner. At the end of the book I've included some items that I think helped me with my healing.

This is my story. I hope you it useful.

Let's Go

You are reading this because you are either where I am, in the process of getting your hip replaced, or contemplating having the procedure. First, congratulations. It is a big decision. I know, I put mine off for ten years. Now I have no choice as the pain is affecting every portion of my life. And I am writing this in real-time, as in, as I write this sentence I am waiting for my scheduled day. I don't know exactly what will happen. I have an idea, but having not experienced it, my knowledge is met with skepticism. Will the pain in my hip really go away? One hundred percent? What's the procedure going to be like? What's the first week like? The second, the third? You get the idea. So I am taking you along for the ride and hopefully provide a trail for you to follow.

I know that you are thirsting for information. And there are some really good places to get good information that go a bit more in-depth than the clinical "What to expect" pages from hospitals and medical pages. The best source, of course, is your doctor. Talk to them. Get personal. After all, this is the person that is going see things only they will see. Your significant other won't even see those things, so don't be shy. I have also found a couple of support groups on Facebook that have been invaluable. Post a question and get almost instant feedback. Feeling down? Put it out there and you will get a flood of support to help you through it. Everybody's journey is different and everyone heals at their own pace, but there is enough commonality that you can get a pretty good idea of what is going on or going to happen. They have been invaluable to me in feeding my hunger for information.

You will find many places to learn what to do before your surgery. From the checklists that the hospital will give you to advice from those who have gone through it so that won't be covered in this book. Not specifically at least — because they will be covered during my preparation, if they're not, I'm sure they will come up in the diary as challenges or frustrations. I'm also not going to tell you what to do, I hope, but to share with you my experience and leave it to you to follow the trail. Good luck on your journey. I hope this peak into my process assists you in yours.

Let's GO!

Crap

It's been years since I was diagnosed with needing this procedure. I've put it off for one reason or another. Mostly out of fear, probably. It's major surgery after all. I'm not good with that. Funny because the damage done came from a lack of fear. A belief that I would be invincible forever… competitive sports, military service, taking the hits and not stopping. That was me. Diving for shots in racquetball. Playing keeper in soccer. Skiing moguls and double black diamond trails. Extreme hiking. Doing everything exciting that I could find during my military career. Go. Go. Go.

What happened?

My first indication that something was wrong came as I was walking up eighth avenue in New York. I had a pain on the outside of my right leg. And for some reason, I just started hitting my hip every few steps with my fist. I thought maybe that something was popping out and when I hit the side of my hip, it felt better. I would learn latter that this is not the preferred method to treat arthritis.

The pain would come and go, and then stay a bit longer. I really wasn't sure what was going on so I made an appointment with my general practitioner who gave me a consult to a senior Orthopedic Surgeon at the same hospital. I got my x-rays and waited patiently with my wife for the doctor to come into the appointment. The clock ticked by. The city below kept its normal pace.

He entered brusquely and took a look at those reversed black and white pictures of my bones.

"Sucks to be forty and need a hip replacement, doesn't it?"

WHAT!!??? What the hell was he talking about? I don't need a replacement… I'll just heal it, I thought.

He pointed to my hip on the screen. "See, here, here, and here. You have almost no cartilage. You have some here, but it's going to shrink."

He had a point.

"How do you think this happened?" He asked.

"I think jumping out of airplanes from extremely high altitude might be bad for your joints," I answered.

"Probably," he said. "Walk for me." He pointed down the hall. I obeyed.

"Yeah, you're shifting your weight. How does it feel?"

"Not too bad," I said. "Is there anything other than surgery that I can do?"

"You can try physical therapy. I'll write you a prescription." He paused for a second and studied the chart again. "The problem is, if you get a replacement now, you'll probably have to get another one in your sixties. Eventually, you'll need to get it replaced."

“Is there anything other than surgery? I'm not sure I want to do that,” I said.

“Not it in the end,” he said. "You might not be ready now. You’ll know when you’re ready. Your body will tell you.” He closed my folder. "But in the end, you're going to need a replacement.”

No I won’t, I thought. I’ll find another way.

There was no other way.

Crap.

Putting It Off

I don't know why I put off the inevitable. Bad advice. A bit of fear. The thought that technology would get better. That maybe I could tough it out. I think in the end it was the bad advice that I should wait ten or so years so that I wouldn't have to have it redone again when I was sixty. Today, technology has progressed to a point where my surgeon thinks the replacement will outlive me. But at the time the replacements had a lifespan of approximately twenty years. When I think back about that advice I get sad. Even if I would have to get the procedure redone at sixty, having a better quality of life for the past decade would have been worth the risk.

There is a lot of fear in the unknown. But putting off a replacement procedure is like not fixing the small water leak — in the end it becomes a huge leak that still needs to be fixed.

∞∞∞

"You cannot escape the responsibility of tomorrow by evading it today." – Abraham Lincoln

WHAT YOU NEED TO KNOW:

Don't put off getting the procedure if you have been diagnosed with needing it done. Get a second opinion. Consult with friends and loved ones. But realize that there is no magic bullet. Any procedure other than the replacement is only a stop-gap until you eventually replace the hip.

24 Days To Go: Final Consult

It's funny how the universe conspires with you in your plans. I didn't want to go back to the surgeon who had first diagnosed me years ago. Partly because I didn't have a great report with him, but mostly because after researching the procedure I wanted to have it done at a hospital the specializes in orthopedic surgery. I wanted to find a surgeon who performed a lot of this type of surgery each year. I wanted to find a place where I felt comfortable.

I thought that it would take a few months to get in to see my top picks. And months after that to get the surgery scheduled, but like the quote attributed to Goethe, "What You Can Do, or Dream You Can, Begin It; Boldness Has Genius, Power, and Magic in It", not only did I just have a great meeting with the surgeon, but the operation is now scheduled to happen in four weeks! There was an option to get it done even earlier, but I didn't think there was enough time to prepare. And I didn't want to feel rushed.

I didn't expect it to come this fast, but maybe it's a good thing — less time to think about the procedure.

∞∞∞

"In preparing for battle I have always found that plans are useless, but planning is indispensable." — Dwight D. Eisenhower

WHAT YOU NEED TO KNOW:
Once you commit to having the procedure done realize that the timeframe might be much different than you originally planned.

21 Days To Go: No, I'm Good

The human mind is a funny thing. Today I woke up with my hip feeling pretty good. So much so that as I poured my coffee a little voice inside my head whispered, "Maybe I don't need surgery yet." This was quickly met with the opposing image of my x-ray that shows bone-on-bone, bone spurs, and a reshaping of the socket. Both sides fighting for control of of my mind like Barnes and Elias in the movie Platoon. It is a conversation that I have had with myself for years and one of the reasons that I have not yet had the THR.

The pain is the devil I know. Recovery is something that I don't. And to be honest this hip has become a part of my identity. Not willfully, but quietly. I walk slower, which in New York is an issue, I'm less sure on my feet, I am no longer active in sports, all negatives in my life, and yet, it has still become who I am. I feel like I am giving up on a piece of myself.

Why are we so resistant to change? Even when that change is good?

The one ray of hope I have since scheduling the surgery, is the fact that the most unfamiliar thought keeps popping into my head — that I could actually feel pain in my hip with the knowledge that it would get better day by day, instead of where I currently am — where I know, day by day it can only get worse. In my mind, for so long, there has been no concept of better. Even with that, I'm scared.

∞∞∞

"You don't concentrate on risks. You concentrate on results. No risk is too great to prevent the necessary job from getting done." — Chuck Yeager

WHAT YOU NEED TO KNOW:

You've lived with this pain and coped with this pain for so long you think that you can just keep doing it forever. You can't. It will continue to get worse and your quality of life will continue to degrade. You need the procedure. Get it done.

20 Days To Go: The Last Hurdle

Yesterday I got my appointment for my class and pre-operation physical, the last hurdle to finally getting this done. And with it, additional stress. I'm in fairly good health, but even so, any time I get a physical I think the worst. What if they find something and I can't go forward with the planned date? It takes a lot to mentally process the fact that you are going to have the surgery. Like getting the nerve to jump off the high dive for the first time, or jump out of an airplane. I'm not sure how I would handle a false start.

∞∞∞

"If you spend too much time thinking about a thing, you'll never get it done." – Bruce Lee

WHAT YOU NEED TO KNOW: Don't freak out about your pre-operation physical. There is no information until you actually have information. Just move forward with the plan until there is no more need to move forward.

17 Days To Go: How Deep The Forest

This weekend I saw a picture of Machu Picchu — a place I have always wanted to go but have thought during the past few years that it was out of reach. No way that I would be able to handle the hikes and climbs. When I saw the picture this weekend there was a little voice in the back of my head that whispered, "you actually might be able to do this yet." It was an interesting feeling, that birth of optimism.

Since getting a date for my surgery, it has constantly been on my mind. The thought does recede into the background when I am doing things, but it is still there with all of its nagging thoughts. Both positive and negative. I am slowly becoming aware that this is major surgery and even though my doc does three-hundred of these a year and that the procedure only takes two hours, it isn't small stuff. It's not getting your wisdom teeth pulled. I've had surgery before, but it was so long ago that I have forgotten the recovery. And now, from slaking my thirst for information, I am waking up. That frightens me. The disruption to my life. The forecast tiredness and stamina issues. The relearning how to use my muscles properly, overcoming the years of compensation. I am trying to keep all of that at arm's length.

When I wrote my first novel I entered the forest blissfully unaware of how deep and dark it was. I pressed on and came out the other side partly because I had no idea how much farther I had to go. My second novel has been a struggle partly because I remember that forest. I fear that I don't know how deep or dark the forest of recovery from this surgery is. All I know is that I will be able to sleep in more than one position again. That I will be able to row without my knee bending outside of my elbow. That I will be able to eventually hike and possibly, quite possibly, get to Machu Picchu.

∞∞∞

"Never measure the height of a mountain until you have reached the top. Then you will see how low it was." - Dag Hammarskjold

WHAT YOU NEED TO KNOW:

Look for information about what you're about to go through, but realize that your path is different. Everyone will heal at their own pace. And just because something happened to someone else, it does not mean it will happen for you. Everyone's forest is a different depth.

15 Days To Go: Houston We Are a Go

All afternoon yesterday, from 1:00PM until 4:30PM, I was in the hospital for pre-screening, medical clearance, and joint replacement class. So much information and apprehension. I am now cleared and that brings with it both excitement and anxiety. I can't believe that within two weeks I will no longer have the pain that I have come to live with for the past several years. That I will be able to again tie my shoes. That I will no longer have that constant ache and constant reminder that I am getting older. The bad hip makes me feel old. That's what I think I hate most about it. And I found yesterday that I have lost height. Probably from the loss of cartilage and the adjustment my pelvis has had to make to accommodate the compensations that I make for the bad hip.

There are a lot of unknowns in this procedure. I have to give credit to the Hospital for Special Surgery for the job that they do in giving the patient the information needed to at least have some idea of what will happen during the journey. It's still academic at this point and not experiential, but it's something to hold on to as the rocket gets prepared.

I take solace in the knowledge of how many people have this procedure done, but still feel like John Glenn on top of the Mercury rocket — I understand what is going to happen, but I have no idea what to expect of the experience.

∞∞∞

"You can't relive your life." - John Glenn

WHAT YOU NEED TO KNOW:

Even with all of the information given to you, you will still feel like there is this big unknown sitting just outside of your vision. This is normal. Only you can go through what you are about to go through. Trust yourself.

14 Days To Go: A Fond Farewell

I am now exactly two weeks out from my surgery. It's amazing how a little time can drastically change something. A good buddy of mine and I met up last night to toast a farewell to my old hip. It was damage honorably inflicted and we felt we should say good bye to a hip that has served me and the country well. I'm kind of attached to it. Pun intended.

I'm trying to not think about the procedure but find that it is always somewhere on my mind. I suppose that's normal. As much as I want to not think this is a big deal, it is major surgery. I can feel my mind and body beginning to get prepared for the journey ahead. When I was in the military, before a mission, there was a period of quiet. A calmness that came over you knowing that you had trained and prepared as much as possible and now it was only up to the execution and to fate. I feel that calmness coming over me now. I just hope this ride is as good as everyone says it is.

∞∞∞

"If all difficulties were known at the outset of a long journey, most of us would never start out at all." - Dan Rather

WHAT YOU NEED TO KNOW:
You will find yourself thinking a lot about your upcoming procedure. Just know that it will end up being entirely different than you think right now.

13 Days To Go: Support Network

Last night was a bit tough. Ever since I have passed all the pre-surgery tests and have gotten the date for the procedure, the idea of the operation has never left my mind. It sometimes fades into the background or sits quietly on the edges of my mind, but it is always there. I posted the same on the support group and immediately received responses, thirty up to date, telling me that they had gone through the exact same thing.

My wife, too, is my biggest champion providing more support than needed, or maybe just the right amount. I don't feel like I need support but obviously, I do. My wife, my friends, and my

Facebook group will be the pillars of my rehabilitation. They will allow me to just be where I need to be, when I need to be there.

∞∞∞

"Life is not a solo act. It's a huge collaboration, and we all need to assemble around us the people who care about us and support us in times of strife." — Tim Gunn

WHAT YOU NEED TO KNOW:

Find your support group. Find your support system. It will be an important part of your healing, both physically and mentally. Remember, this is a major procedure. Or so, everyone keeps reminding me.

12 Days To Go: Getting Prepared

With two weekends left before my procedure I am now beginning to get things prepared… Make sure there is enough freezer space for the ice bags, etc. Still not sure if I am going to use frozen peas or the compression cold therapy pants. Not sure if one works better than the other. They both need constant attention to the ice. Also looking at reclining chairs today. A lot of people swear by them on the support group page. It really won't fit into a New York apartment, but I think we can deal with the cramped space for the comfort it will provide.

The pain seems to be getting even worse. Maybe my hip knows that I am planning on replacing it and it's now making itself even more known. Or, it might be like when you buy a car of a certain color, all you see are cars of that color. Maybe I'm so focused on the operation that my thoughts are always on my hip and pain that I would have previously ignored is now front and center in my mind.

∞∞∞

"It is thrifty to prepare today for the wants of tomorrow." — Aesop

WHAT YOU NEED TO KNOW:

Make sure your house is prepared for when you come home from the hospital. Your known universe is going to be what you can see around you right now. So, have frozen meals ready. Ice ready. Make sure you have the tools you will need to allow yourself to heal.

11 Days To Go: A New Fear

Over this weekend my wife and I went shopping for a recliner to assist in the rest portion of my healing formula. So many options. So many price-points. Part of me feels guilty in spending the money on comfort, but I also know that that thought is ridiculous.

I also emailed my doctor as to which implant I am getting. I wish I hadn't have done that as it led me down the rabbit hole of internet health advice. Every recall of every hip type came up in the search. This is really too much information for me to know. I am an advocate for knowing all there is to know about my procedure, but I am not in a position to judge which implant is best. That is the job of my orthopedic surgeon. My job was to select the right surgeon. Now my job is done and I need to trust in his skill and prescription.

∞∞∞

"The time to take counsel of your fears is before you make an important battle decision. That's the time to listen to every fear you can imagine! When you have collected all the facts and fears and made your decision, turn off all your fears and go ahead!" — George S. Patton

WHAT YOU NEED TO KNOW:
Don't read too much information on the internet. Interact with your support group. Read some case studies so you know what to expect during your recovery. But do not over think the process and the surgery. All you will see are the monsters in the shadows and that is a stress your body doesn't need prior to your surgery.

10 Days To Go: A Reminder

Last night was really bad. Extreme pain. And yesterday I made the mistake of looking into all of the possible side effects and things that could go wrong with the operation. I started to have thoughts of staying with the devil you know rather than the angel you don't. That maybe my pain was still just an annoyance. That's the trick the mind plays. But then came last night and today. Stark reminders that no, the pain is not just an annoyance, that the pain is life restricting and real. A reminder needed to begin preparation for my procedure in ten days. I am both excited and anxious. Excited in thinking that this upcoming weekend will be the last one that I feel that deep, aching, pain and lack of motion in my hip. By next weekend I will be part titanium and can begin to heal.

∞∞∞

"Courage doesn't always roar. Sometimes courage is the little voice at the end of the day that says I'll try again tomorrow." ~Mary Anne Radmacher

WHAT YOU NEED TO KNOW:
When you're questioning your decision to have this procedure take a moment to reflect on the worst pain you have had in your hip. That will soon be gone. It will be replaced by a pain that is temporary and that will lessen day by day as you heal.

09 Days To Go: A New Hope

Today as I put my sock on the bad leg, through my patented method of hooking by ankle behind the calf of the good leg and lifting the foot of my bad leg up towards my left hand, which then swings the sock down to catch my big toe whereby I can then pull the sock up my ankle, I realized that at some point in the future I will no longer need to do this. That I will, once again, be able to put on socks normally. Be able to tie shoes again. Be able to bend over without sticking my bad leg out behind me.

It's amazing the coping mechanisms we come up with isn't it? But all of these give me a new hope.

No longer the thought that it will only continue to get worse. That this pain and lack of mobility is now my lot in life. But the hope that in three weeks the pain and weakness will be the bottom plateau and that with work it can only improve.

We all need hope in our life. For anything. The lack of hope is the beginning of death.

∞∞∞

"Infuse your life with action. Don't wait for it to happen. Make it happen. Make your own future. Make your own hope. Make your own love. And whatever your beliefs, honor your creator, not by passively waiting for grace to come down from upon high, but by doing what you can to make grace happen... yourself, right now, right down here on Earth." — Bradley Whitford

WHAT YOU NEED TO KNOW:

Once you make the decision to move for your will find a new sense of hope. Use that hope. It's a different mindset than the one you've been dealing with during your painful days.

07 Days To Go: Doubts

The weather today matches my mood, which is damp and raining. I've been experiencing some doubt and second guessing as I get closer to the date. It's understandable. It's deep. It's primal. As bad as the pain is, as old as it makes me feel even at a young age, as slow as I move, I can still move. But this surgery will hobble me for a few days, maybe even for a few weeks. And that's frightening. To voluntarily take away the ability to fight or flight and to release your care to the rest of your tribe is a huge decision. I don't do well with letting people help me. The thought of being a burden, for even a short time, makes me uncomfortable. But the facts are the facts. At this point I will never get better. If I don't do the surgery, my hip will degrade to the point of being frozen.

I guess I can take two weeks of helplessness for the ability to regain my strength and again feel my age.

∞∞∞

"I must not fear. Fear is the mind-killer. Fear is the little-death that brings total obliteration. I will face my fear. I will permit it to pass over me and through me. And when it has gone past I will turn the inner eye to see its path. Where the fear has gone there will be nothing. Only I will remain." — Frank Herbert, Dune

WHAT YOU NEED TO KNOW:
Up until the day after surgery you will be questioning your decision. Just remember, if the pain was at such a state that you contemplated the procedure, then your decision to have the procedure done was the correct one. You made

that decision in a state of calm. You are now in a state of anxiety which sows the seeds of doubt.

06 Days To Go: Humor

Yesterday I made a post to my Facebook support group that read, "I've told my wife that mint chocolate chip ice cream is required for proper healing - Not sure she's buying it." It received a hundred reactions and more than fifty comments in support of my claim. Everything from "icing the inside as well as the outside" (suspicious), to "the calcium is good for the bone growth" (plausible). It seems that we all, at whatever stage we are at in this process, need humor to take our minds off of the procedure.

For me, currently, it's not easy to laugh as the operation and all of the possible side effects and outcomes are on my mind. "What if the leg remains longer? Or shorter? Will my bursitis go away? Will my body accept the titanium implant? How long will recovery take?" But I force myself to laugh and it works. I have to remember that this procedure will make my life better. There is only a 3%-4% complication rate. For major surgery those are pretty good odds. I need to keep the stress to a minimum now, going into the final week… need to be happy in body and mind so that my body is ready for the healing that will come.

When I was in the military once the plans of an operation where completed, once they were understood, once the training was deemed complete, once everyone had internalized what was going to happen, then we let loose. We kept ourselves busy with things we enjoyed where we were active so that we didn't overthink the mission. That is what I plan for this next week. Once the house is ready. Once everything is in order I am going to stop thinking about the upcoming procedure. It's Memorial Day weekend here in the U.S. I'm going to pay tribute to those colleagues of mine that were lost and then go have a hot dog in the sun.

∞∞∞

"Like a welcome summer rain, humor may suddenly cleanse and cool the earth, the air and you." — Langston Hughes

WHAT YOU NEED TO KNOW:

Once you have prepared your environment for your return after surgery, live life. Have fun. Laugh. Forget about the upcoming procedure and enjoy the days.

02 Days To Go: Emotions Run High

A long Memorial Day weekend and emotions are starting to run high. Part of it is the deadline of getting everything ready before the big day. There is always something more to do, isn't there? I'm trying not to get too stressed out.

The operation is more in the forefront of my mind now. It feels remarkably like the first time I jumped off the high dive. You watch as your friends all do it and come out of the pool fine and you know that it's safe as long as you don't belly flop, and even then you will just be red for a bit, but you climb the ladder and look over the edge and you hesitate. You don't really know what to expect. You know that gravity will pull you towards the water at an increasing speed and that the water is deep, but you don't really know until you make that jump. I am currently standing on the edge of that platform and in my mind, I am going through everything that can happen. Will my femur fracture? How bad will the pain be in the weeks after. What if something happens during the operation.

It's a difficult time. The only thing I can say to you is to just embrace all of those thoughts and feelings and then just let them go knowing that there have been many people who too have stood on the edge of that high dive and looked over the edge wondering what it will REALLY be like.

∞∞∞

"When dealing with people, remember you are not dealing with creatures of logic, but creatures of emotion." – Dale Carnegie

WHAT YOU NEED TO KNOW:

You will become increasingly emotional in the time leading up to surgery. Know that and treat yourself accordingly. Know that the filter you are seeing things through is temporary.

01 Day To Go: The Day Before

The only thing I have to say today has been said better before…

Lose this day loitering—'twill be the same story To-morrow–and the next more dilatory; Then indecision brings its own delays, And days are lost lamenting o'er lost days. Are you in earnest? seize this very minute–

What you can do, or dream you can, begin it, Boldness has genius, power, and magic in it, Only engage, and then the mind grows heated— Begin it, and the work will be completed!

— From John Anster's translation of Johann Wolfgang von Goethe's Faust.

WHAT YOU NEED TO KNOW:

It's time to go. Boldness has genius, power, and magic in it…

Day Zero: Procedure Day

Yesterday was one of the worst days for pain I have ever had. I had to leave the New York City FC match at the half because I couldn't get comfortable. Sleeping was almost impossible. A part of my thinks it's my body reminding me how bad I need this surgery. Or the universe taking away any doubt. Strange to come the night before my procedure. Especially when I couldn't take anything for the pain.

I'm dressed. I've got everything ready to go. Nothing left but to get this done. My biggest concern right now are blood clots. I feel like I'm on the roller coaster climbing that first big hill to the top of the drop.

Update: I didn't think I'd get time to write an entry this evening. It's now 9:00PM and I've come out the other side. Everything today from admission until ending up here in my room has been super smooth. Arrived at the hospital twelve hours ago and was met by the friendliest admitting crew that I could have imagined. Everything was explained in great detail and the paperwork was organized and quick. Then it was up to the family lounge where my wife would be waiting for updates. I think she had the tougher part of the journey as I just took a nap all day while she had to wait while keeping herself distracted. Not much time to think… they called my name and I was off — Back to pre-op where my vitals were checked, my IV's inserted, the area prepped and I got to meet all the people that would be on my team.

And then — It's time! They wheel me to the hallway and I kiss my wife as we come to the time to part. She, off to the waiting room, and me into the operating wing. The first thing I notice is how cold it is… which makes sense as it helps keep down infection and the operating teams are all in their moon suits.

My operating room is almost at the end of the hall so I get to go by each of the rooms along the way. Inside I see blue-clad teams huddled around metal tables hard at work. The orderlies I pass on my way to my OR all smile and wish me well. It's comforting and I feel like I'm entering a sporting arena.

The room is not really what I expected. Bigger with more stations than I imagined. There is a cart with at least one hundred devices, gleaming, and ready for action. It reminds me of an automotive shop. It's the last thought I have before I drift off to sleep.

I alternate waking and drifting back off to sleep in recovery. Once awake I get interviewed by my recovery nurse to assess my status and check my vitals. It's now around 4:30 and I'm offered an Italian ice. It's the best thing I've ever had.

∞∞∞

"Sometimes we should express our gratitude for the small and simple things like the scent of the rain, the taste of your favorite food, or the sound of a loved one's voice." — Joseph B. Wirthlin

WHAT YOU NEED TO KNOW:

You did the work in choosing the surgeon. Now it's time to trust them to do what they do best. You're going to be fine.

Day 01 PO: Sleeping Without Pain

First good night's sleep in a very long time. Up every few hours, but the sleep I did get was deep and pain free. Some of that is due to the drugs but also due to the fact that my hip is fixed. My muscles this morning feel like I hiked five miles, but no pain in the hip. I can feel that it's there and I can feel that I had an operation, but I'm comfortable. Pain scale a 1-2 instead of an 8-9.

∞∞∞

"Take rest; a field that has rested gives a beautiful crop." — Ovid

WHAT YOU NEED TO KNOW:

That deep pain that you have lived with for so long—the pain that you had learned to endure—will now be gone. Enjoy the feeling. It's like hearing music for the first time.

Day 03 PO: Coming Home

Today was all a bit of a happy blur. Being released from the hospital I am now ensconced in my recliner with ice and a cool drink. Yesterday my physical therapist had me walk my required two laps around the ward and then prove that I could climb the set of stairs without too much difficulty. Once that milestone was reached I was marked cleared for departure. Out of the hospital gown and into my sweats!

My goal was to leave with only a cane; having a walker in a New York City apartment is a bit of an impediment. Fortunately, I am walking well enough that no walker was needed. I don't know where we would have stored the thing anyway. I have a strange clicking feel when I walk. The surgeon says that it's normal—apparently the tendons are popping a bit as I walk. Feels weird, and I still feel a bit wobbly, but I can report that the deep bone-on-bone pain is gone. Or maybe that's the pain medication talking.

Coming home was a bit of an ordeal. It was a bit of a challenge getting into the passenger side of the car and the ride home was a bit uncomfortable. I don't think that I've ever noticed how many potholes there are in New York. I closed my eyes, took deep breaths, and hoped I was ready for my next test. My biggest concern were the thirty stairs I needed to climb to get to our apartment. I shouldn't have been. With the cane and the railing all was fine, although I did have the pleasant thought that I wouldn't have to do that again for at least a couple of days.

I've got my books, my iPad, my cold therapy machine, and my wife. It's good to be home. Let the healing begin!

∞∞∞

"There is nothing like staying at home for real comfort." — Jane Austen

WHAT YOU NEED TO KNOW:

You're going to feel wobbly. You're going to feel vulnerable. But you're going to be fine. Coming home is your first test out in the real world. Be careful with your 90 degree restriction. Take your time and don't let anyone rush you. And relish the fact that you're home. You made it home.

Day 04 PO: Gratitude

Today is day four, post-op, and I am, I don't know if I can describe this correctly, awash in a feeling of gratitude. The only pain in my body is in the muscles of my right leg and butt and that has even abated a bit. We don't know, when we are living with chronic pain, how much it affects ALL of the systems of our body. This morning as I sit and take an inventory of how my body feels, there is a general calm. Like the storm has passed. I imagine a meadow after a summer shower. Water still drips from the leaves of milkweed plants and the clouds in the sky are broken with shards of blue appearing in the empty spaces. It's a good place to be.

There is so much gratitude for all of those who have helped me through this journey; those of who

I was aware and those of who I wasn't. From the nurses who watched over me at night to the Uber driver who consciously tried to avoid the pot holes and dips of the New York City street landscape to minimize the bumps. My surgeon and the surgical team. The orderlies who wished me luck on my way to the operating theater and the recovery nurses who guided me out of the woods of sedation.

∞∞∞

"Gratitude, warm, sincere, intense, when it takes possession of the bosom, fills the soul to overflowing and scarce leaves room for any other sentiment or thought."
— John Quincy Adams

WHAT YOU NEED TO KNOW:
Once you make it through the procedure you be amazed at what your body had become accustomed to — the absence of pain is like experiencing the silence of the country after living in the city for years.

Day 05 PO: Clothes Make The Man

Today I am in my new uniform. Loose fitting gym shorts and a t-shirt. Yesterday it was warm-up pants and a t-shirt. Tomorrow it will be more of the same. I am not winning any awards for fashion but the only one who sees me now are my wife, the physical therapist, and the nurse who is keeping tabs on my incision. I think they're okay with my choice of clothes.

Before the operation my wife and I went to the store and stocked up on this style of clothing. I won't be able to wear jeans for another couple of weeks. The incision is right were the thick seem of the jeans hit your leg. I can wait two weeks… until then I'll just pretend I'm training for the Olympics.

∞∞∞

"Clothes make the man. Naked people have little or no influence on society." — Mark Twain

WHAT YOU NEED TO KNOW:

Make sure you have clothes that are loose fitting and comfortable. There cannot be too much pressure on the incision. Don't worry… few people are going to see you anyways.

Day 06 PO: Shawshank

Today for PT my therapist added going outside to the regular exercises. This is a major deal in NYC as I now have to contend with uneven surfaces, other pedestrians, and dogs. I've just noticed that everyone seems to have a dog. With my wife and the therapist as blockers for those coming behind, I tentatively left the apartment and turned onto the sidewalk. The world again seems so large. The thought of going across to ninth avenue seems overwhelming. But I'm out. For the first time since returning from the hospital I can feel the sun on my face. My view is more than the inside of my living room. And now for the big event… crossing the street. Not once, but four times. I know, something we all learned to do at age six or seven is now a big deal. Timing is everything. I wait until the light changes and then go… A step down off the curb, just like the stairs, except due to the increased stimuli — people, traffic, etc., I forget to lead with the cane and operated leg. Across I go to pause and prepare for the next. And then the next. And finally the last. Success! Four crossings and I'm still alive. Now, back upstairs to ice.

∞∞∞

"The secret to happiness is freedom… And the secret to freedom is courage." — Thucydides

WHAT YOU NEED TO KNOW:
Take the risks. Force your body to grow. I learned in the military that we are capable of so much more physically than we actually think we are. The largest factor of endurance is mental. Release the shackles and heal.

Day 09 PO: Pain Returns

Yesterday during a check of my vitals my physical therapist noticed that my pulse was skipping occasionally. This, of course, was disconcerting. A quick search of the Google — the worst doctor available — put my mind at ease. Palpitations are a side effect of oxycodone. Pretty common too, which is disappointing as I always want to be far from common. So I didn't take any doses prior to going to sleep.

My pain level this morning is double of what it was. Fortunately, I was doing really well so now my pain is only moderate. I feel now things that were masked. My back hurts a bit. I can feel the ache deep in my thigh…I imagine that that is the implant cementing itself into my bone as my body starts to heal around it. I have aches around my hip that are echoes of my arthritis and the bursitis. This is disappointing as I was enjoying the feeling of nothing where there used to be pain. It's not as sharp and deep as it was pre-surgery, but there is something there.

∞∞∞

"When things are a disappointment, try not to be so discouraged." — Carol Burnett

WHAT YOU NEED TO KNOW:
The pain medication takes away more pain than you realize. Don't be disappointed with the return of pain. You have just had a major procedure and are healing. But even the pain of recovery is far less than the pain you experienced before the operation.

Day 12 PO: Nap Like A Cat

My days now tend to follow the same pattern. Wake up and take my pills, which need thirty minutes before eating, do my first round of exercises, shower, eat breakfast, and retire to my recliner and my best friend, the cold therapy machine. I've frozen water bottles to use with water instead of ice and each set lasts about five hours.

Wake up, walk around, eat, nap, walk around, nap, walk around, eat, read, nap some more. I have found myself tired, but not in a bad way but in a "my body is building new tissue and needs you to shut down for a little while" kind of way. Napping is good. I imagine that this is the life of a golden retriever. I would write more, but it's time for my nap.

∞∞∞

"Rest when you're weary. Refresh and renew yourself, your body, your mind, your spirit. Then get back to work." — Ralph Marston

WHAT YOU NEED TO KNOW:
You are going to nap. A lot! This is good. Do not feel guilty about it. The body needs rest to heal just as much as it needs the exercise. Don't be a hero. Take your pain meds, work out, and nap.

Day 16 PO: Ups And Downs

Today was a bad day. From going along smoothly, ticking all of the check boxes and moving forward, today felt like I had regressed. My PT tells me that it's a combination of reducing my pain medication, some nerves coming back on line, and some swelling going down. I can tell that the pain is muscular and not that deep bone pain before the surgery and that makes me happy. It's all perspective. Before the operation pain meant degradation and the slow erosion of my quality of life. Pain now means recovery and another step up the hill to getting my life back. It is still frustrating as hell.

∞∞∞

"Temporary setbacks are overshadowed by persistence." – Quentin L. Cook

WHAT YOU NEED TO KNOW:
It's not going to be all forward progress. There will be times where your body just doesn't want to work for you. It's frustrating, but normal. Press on.

Day 19 PO: It's A Small World

Wow. It's amazing how small your world feels when the furthest points are dictated by how far you can walk and the lack of endurance. Currently my radius is one long city block in either direction or three to four short blocks. My known universe has contracted to my recliner and apartment with short jaunts out into the world. I have no idea what is going on in my neighborhood, my city, or the places that I used to frequent. All that is known is all that I can see.

∞∞∞

"Always remember your focus determines your reality." - George Lucas

WHAT YOU NEED TO KNOW:
You will feel restricted and small and vulnerable. This is normal. Remember that this is the time where you should be focusing on healing your hip. Ice. Rest. Heal. Your world will get big again, I promise.

Day 21 PO: Humility

As adults we tend to forget how independent we really are. We take it for granted. The ability to go where you want, when you want, is given to us late in our teens or early twenties. It's something we're used to. Now, three weeks out, it is luxurious to be escorted to a cafe a long New York City block away and left to my own devices. One of the biggest things I've had to deal with is allowing myself to be dependent. To, if even for a short time, require most of my needs to be assisted in some manner. It doesn't make you feel weak, per se, just smaller. And a realization dawns about the fragility of man. And an empathy for those growing old who rapidly find themselves not as independent as they once were. I feel like a child again where key milestones are being met. Can I cross the street? Can I go out on my own? How far from the apartment can I travel? Can I cook dinner? In short if left alone, could I survive?

∞∞∞

"It's not a bad idea to occasionally spend a little time thinking about things you take for granted. Plain everyday things." — Evan Davis

WHAT YOU NEED TO KNOW:

Your support person is the most important tool in your arsenal. Make sure you have a good network before you go in for your procedure. They will make the healing faster and easier.

Day 27 PO: Learning To Walk Again

As I walked away from my physical therapist so that he could evaluate how I was walking, I realized that this is probably going to be the biggest challenge—learning how to walk properly again. The human body is an amazingly adaptable piece of art. When a portion isn't working properly, like my hip, weight shifts, muscles compensate, and tendons adjust. After five really bad years I have forgotten how to walk as I was designed.

It's the physical therapist's job to not let you cheat. To not let you compensate. And it's hard. It hurts. But unlike the pain of the arthritis prior to the operation, this pain lessens a bit day by day.

∞∞∞

"The rewards for those who persevere far exceed the pain that must precede the victory." — Ted Engstrom

WHAT YOU NEED TO KNOW:

Your muscles have atrophied. Your tendons have shortened. Your center of balance is off. You will be able to fix all this within a relatively short time so don't get discouraged, just press on.

Six Weeks

Today was my six week check up with the surgeon. Wow! Six weeks. It only feels like a year.

One of my goals before this started was to be able to make it from my apartment to my appointment free of my cane. This is a somewhat frightening proposition, given the shifting of the subway, the steps, etc. Two weeks ago, I was able to attend the NYCFC match so I had a pretty good idea that I would make my goal. Because of my PT team, today I dressed in shorts and tennis shoes and was able to arrive at my surgeon's office, cane free.

I got cleared of the 90 degree restrictions and am allowed back into the pool and was told to come back in another six weeks. That everything was exactly what they hope to see. It's the first time that I've seen the x-ray of my new hip. Seeing it in person I've decided to name him — Hippy McHipster, or Ti for short. He is made of Titanium to be fair…

It's good to have goals. But I have to remind myself to not be so focused on my goals that I cheat or compensate in other ways to reach them. Justin, my physical therapist, has been pretty good at keeping me honest. Painfully so. And with each new victory, riding the stationary bike, balancing on the balance board for thirty seconds or more, or increasing weight on the leg press, I know that I am getting the solid foundation to continue until I'm back at one-hundred percent.

∞∞∞

"Successful people maintain a positive focus in life no matter what is going on around them. They stay focused on their past successes rather than their past failures, and on the next action steps they need to take to get them closer to the fulfillment of their goals rather

than all the other distractions that life presents to them."

— Jack Canfield

WHAT YOU NEED TO KNOW:

Set goals. Achieve your goals. But don't be disappointed if you don't. Know that your goals are supposed to be at the edge of possibility.

Ten Weeks

There are flashes of brilliance. I'll be walking down the street and realize that I have no pain. No forceful exhale of breath on each painful step. It actually feels good to walk. Freeing. Like I could walk forever and anywhere. Then there are days when I feel the familiar pain from before the surgery. Not the arthritis, that's gone, but the tendinitis down the inner thigh, the groin pain from the hip flexor, the weakness of the core muscles. This is all pain that can be healed, but I am surprised at its persistence. I shouldn't be. For ten years those muscles and tendons were misused because of the lack in range in motion. The pain I was feeling then was for the same reasons now, except then there was not much I could do about it.

I had envisioned my time after surgery to be pain free and full of rainbows and unicorns, but it's not. It's a process. And I have to remind myself that it was only ten weeks ago that that part of my body went through major trauma. Ten weeks will not erase ten years. But I'm on my way.

∞∞∞

"The most essential factor is persistence - the determination never to allow your energy or enthusiasm to be dampened by the discouragement that must inevitably come." — James Whitcomb Riley

WHAT YOU NEED TO KNOW:
You will have good days and bad. Days that you feel you can conquer anything and days where you feel pain and remember the time before surgery. Remember that you are still healing. It will take up to a year to be fully healed.

Twenty Weeks

I thought I would be further along by now. Don't get me wrong, I've been cleared by my surgeon until the year anniversary, have been fly fishing again, am walking without pain most days, but I wanted to be able to tie my shoes in a normal manner by now. I wanted to be totally pain free and not fighting occasionally with my hip flexor and IT band.

Apparently, it is all normal. The swelling deep inside doesn't fully go away for six months and it took a lot of years for my hip flexor and IT band to get into the shape they were in, it's going to take a long time for me to get them back into proper shape.

All in all, it's good. Before I had the procedure when I'd speak to others who had had it done who said that it was the best decision they ever made, I thought that it was hyperbole. But looking back, I can say it's not. It was one of the best decisions I ever made. Before the surgery I felt older. With each step, the pain would remind me that my hip was deteriorating. I would look at activities I once participated in and feel nostalgic. Going to a movie and cooping with being uncomfortable for two hours became too much. Travel, one of the great joys of my life, had become hard. Sitting in an airline seat for five or more hours became almost unbearable. My range when walking around new cities had been reduced by at least half. Now, twenty weeks later, I feel like myself again. My walking radius is back to that of a proper New Yorker. I am no longer concerned about how far or what type of streets I'll be walking. In short I got my life back and now my only regret is that I waited as long as I did.

∞∞∞

"Transformation is a process, and as life happens there are tons of ups and downs. It's a journey of discovery

- there are moments on mountaintops and moments in deep valleys of despair." — Rick Warren

WHAT YOU NEED TO KNOW:

Everything that you heard is true. It's a major operation. There are risks. But in the end the reward is worth the risk.

A Look Back

When I started this journey there were a lot of unknowns. I didn't know what the operation would be like. I didn't know what the recovery would be like. I was fearful of infection. I was fearful of the unknowns. Looking back I had been afraid for a long time.

Once the pain made the decision for me and I had to face my fears it took a lot of energy. As you can tell, it has been a bit of an emotional roller coaster. Ten years ago when my doctor first diagnosed my arthritis and prescribed surgery, I balked. He then said what I now know to be the wisest words yet — "You'll know when you're ready."

I wish I had been ready earlier, but maybe there are reasons why I wasn't. We all get here at our own pace. And we all heal at our own pace. Remember that.

Some benefits that have come from having the procedure done:

- My blood pressure has returned to levels from five years ago.
- My friends tell me I look happy again. That scowl that had found a home on my face is now gone.
- I've lost a few pounds. Since I can again walk I can do more than just swim at the gym.
- My knee pain has gone away. I had shifted my balance so much that other joints were started to become affected.
- My bursitis is gone.
- My grace is back. I have balance again.

- I have joy when I walk. The simple act of walking down the street, pain free, brings me unbelievable joy.

Was it hard? Yes. Was it scary? Yes.

Would I do it again? Yes.

I wish you well where ever you are on the timeline of this journey. May your outcome be as positive as mine has been.

Peace.

Tips and Notes

I have been extremely fortunate. Either by genetics, my surgeon's skill, or luck, I have had a fairly easy recovery. On my birthday, eight weeks and four days post op, I spent the day by driving for over an hour, taking a boat to a small island in Long Island Sound, hiking around the island through soft sand, uneven terrain, a rock sea wall, up and down hills, and swimming in the sound. I still had to ice when I came home, and I still had pain in the tendons, but it was improvement. I have also spent a week in the Adirondacks, driven twelve hours to watch the solar eclipse, and have frequently logged more than 15,000 steps on my Garmin. I'm a new man.

Please remember that everyone heals AT THEIR OWN PACE and that's okay. There are many factors that come into play. I would like to think that some of how I approached my healing is one of the reasons for my fast recovery, so I want to include them here in the hope that them might help you as well.

Remember that healing is in large part a mental activity. You need to give your body permission to heal. I don't mean in a hocus pocus way, I mean in a very specific manner. When I was in the military I had to go through an extremely physical test that lasts for over twelve hours. Its purpose is to push you to where you THINK your physical limit is and then push you beyond, to show you that getting through anything physical is 80% mental. I used that knowledge to help my body through this ordeal, and it is an ordeal, don't let others tell you otherwise. I set goals. I wanted to leave the hospital with a cane and not a walker. I wanted to be able to go to a sporting event with a large crowd in my fourth week. I wanted to go to my six week surgeon review without a cane. And I wanted to be able to jog a bit by my birthday in week eight… I didn't make that last one. It's a bit crazy but you get the idea.

Rest and allow your body to heal. Give yourself permission to nap and sleep late. And take your pain medication. This is no time to be heroic. Your body is building new bone and soft tissue. That will take a toll. Don't feel lazy because you need to behave like a dog or cat during the day. My goal for the first week was to be like a golden retriever. Wake up, eat, walk around a little bit, do my PT, take a nap, wake up, move a little bit, nap, eat a little more, nap, etc. I strongly believe that the speed of my recovery was that I laid a foundation during the first two weeks of doing the absolute minimum possible. Yes, do your PT exercises — that is paramount, but other than that, it was ice and nap. That gave my body the time to heal so when I was ready to start pushing the boundaries, it was ready.

Eat nutrient dense foods. Give your body the fuel it needs to do what it needs to do. During my recovery, I made sure that I included nutrient dense foods in my diet. I adjusted my purple smoothie to take out the foods that would interact with my medication, like turmeric, which is a blood thinner, and cinnamon, which is an anti-inflammatory. I made sure that I ate three meals a day and that I drank plenty of water.

Do your physical therapy, but remember that you are the boss. Do what your physical therapist tells you to do but remember that it's your body and that you are the boss. If something feels wrong, tell the PT and don't do it. Only you can feel what is going on. If you feel that you can do one more set, tell them and do so. You don't want to over extend yourself, but you do want to let your body do what it can. Some of what you feel is normal and they will tell you, remember your muscles have a lot of relearning to do and your leg has been manipulated pretty roughly to get that new hip into place, but sometimes you're just not ready to move forward. On a day off from PT I went for my daily walk, I pushed it a bit too far probably and got a slight pull in my hamstring. I iced it right away and the next day told the PT that I would need to take it easy during the session. They adjusted accordingly and everything went back on track.

Ice, ice, baby. Ice will be your best friend. Ice will take away the pain you will feel, reduce the swelling, and help you heal. The best pre-op decision I made was to purchase a cold therapy machine which circulates cold water through a pad that you wear on your hip, and a recliner which allowed me to rest comfortably without breaking the 90 degree restriction. If you get a cold therapy machine, remember this hack… the instructions tell you to fill the reservoir with water and then ice, but you can avoid the hassle of refilling with ice every five-to-six hours if you use frozen water bottles. My machine held four eight ounce bottles, so we used a method of freezing twelve bottles. Four were in the machine, four were being refrozen from the last use, and four were ready to go. You just swap out the bottles and you're good to go. I believe that this machine and the constant icing was one of the biggest contributors to my rapid recovery.

Allow yourself to fail. As much as I wanted to push myself — I'm a bit of an overachiever — I also knew that there would be things that I would want to do but couldn't. Things that others might be able to do at my stage in recovery but couldn't. Yes, I would get frustrated, but would then remember rule number one… Everyone heals at their own pace. My body was going to fail. But it would not fail forever. That each failure was triggering the muscles to become stronger. So I accepted the failure, internalized it, and let it go. I was where I was and really, after all I had put my body through, could I really ask for more? You have gone through major surgery. It's a major trauma to the body. The body has to adjust to the new reality. I have had to again find my center of balance as over the past five years my body shifted that balance over the good hip and leg, muscles and tendons need to come back to life after not being used properly, and your heart and soul need time to adjust to the fact that the pain you feel is no longer the degeneration of your hip and the constant loss of motion, but the strengthening and healing of your new hip and your body reclaiming its ability to move properly.

∞∞∞

Tools:

Cold therapy machine. There are many out there, some are covered by insurance, especially if you rent from a medical supply store. I didn't want to rent as that would only last two weeks and for cheaper than my co-pay I could purchase my own from Amazon. I purchased the Ossur Cold Therapy Machine. You should make your own choice, but I swear by this one.

Recliner: If you have one, great. If you can buy or rent one, do. I live in a New York apartment and I know how space can be limited. This was a purchase that made the first two weeks possible. One note, however, is not to sleep in the recliner for more than one or two nights. Your body needs to stretch and relax on a flat surface and you need to raise your feet above your heart to help reduce the swelling.

Social Media: Look at the Total Hip Replacement groups on Facebook and join a few. These groups have been invaluable to me as a place to commune with people who have gone through or are going through the same thing you are. Only someone who has had this procedure knows exactly what you are going through emotionally and physically.

Physical Therapy: I've heard that some doctors don't prescribe this, and I can't imagine why. If your insurance allows for PT, use it. It has been the one resource to ensure that I am using proper mechanics in my exercises. As different muscles come back online, the body will want to compensate. As you regain your balance and grace, you need these checkpoints to maximize your healing.

Purple Smoothie: If you have a blender that can make smoothies there is no need to go out and buy something new. If you don't, I use the Nutra Ninja. Here's the recipe for pre-op and post-op and the one for after you are off all medication.

1 banana
1 cup frozen blueberries
1/2 cup frozen pineapple
1 cup frozen kale or kale/spinach mix
2 Tbs chia seeds
2 Tbs cocoa nibs (It's important to use raw nibs. This is not chocolate, but the base of chocolate and contains fiber, iron, and magnesium.)
2 cups almond, soy, or other nut milk. More or less depending on how thick you like your smoothie.

After you are off of medications you can add the following. (Check with your doctor first.)

1tsp fresh ginger
1tsp fresh or ground turmeric
1tsp cinnamon

The smoothie will last in the refrigerator for twenty-four hours. Although it will turn from purple to green due to the chlorophyll in the spinach and kale. And don't worry, you don’t taste the kale.

∞∞∞

Good luck!

One Last Word

It has been said many times in this book and you will hear it over and over — we all heal at our pace. Your experience will be different from mine. Maybe by a little, maybe by a lot. It was my goal to provide some trail markers and share my experience as beacon to follow and hopefully provide some calm.

If you got something out of this book, please leave a review or share with others you know who are about to become hippies. And stop by www.diaryofahippie.com and let everyone know how you're doing!

You've got this!

About The Author

John lives in New York with his wife and is the author of articles, short fiction, and novels. He is an incurable wanderlust and is currently working on the novel The Heart.

To contact John, please use the contact form on his site, www.johnharbour.com.

Follow John:
Twitter: @John_Harbour
Facebook: AuthorJohnHarbour
Medium: @John_Harbour

CPSIA information can be obtained
at www.ICGtesting.com
Printed in the USA
FFOW02n1116031217
43820720-42751FF